Table of Contents

Introduction

As more Americans are affected by poor diet choices, chronic stress, toxic overload and bacterial imbalance, it appears that the prevalence of leaky gut is potentially reaching epidemic proportions. The medical profession is just now agreeing this condition even exists, which is especially shocking considering that "intestinal permeability" (another name for leaky gut) has been discussed in the medical literature for over 100 years!

Why should leaky gut syndrome concern you? In recent years, studies consider leaky gut a "danger signal for autoimmune disease."

Below is a brief description of common leaky gut syndrome symptoms seen in people struggling with this condition. A four-step process is recommended to help promote healing including trigger foods to remove from your diet and beneficial supplements to add in.

Leaky gut syndrome (or intestinal permeability) is a condition that affects the lining of the intestines. This can result in symptoms like persistent muscle or joint pain, poor concentration, indigestion, gas, mood swings, nervousness, skin rashes, recurrent bladder or yeast infections, constipation, or anxiety.

However, there is no scientific data in humans that a leaky gut resulting in increased intestinal permeability causes symptoms outside the gastrointestinal (GI) tract. Leaky gut syndrome is considered a theory, rather than a condition traditionally recognized by the general medical community.

Symptoms of Leaky Gut

It's important to note that symptoms of a "leaky gut" are nonspecific, meaning they can be caused by many other conditions. Symptoms attributed to leaky gut syndrome may include the following:

- Bloating
- Abdominal discomfort
- Diarrhea
- Constipation
- Fatigue
- Skin rashes
- Joint pain
- Headaches

Because the symptoms overlap with other conditions, evaluation requires a workup by your healthcare provider to exclude other causes.

What Causes Leaky Gut?

Like the skin, the gastrointestinal (GI) tract, which is the digestive tube that runs from the mouth to the anus, is continuously exposed to external substances. It requires a specialized layer of defense to prevent the random passage of bacteria and toxins into the body.

This barrier defense includes a mucus layer, an epithelial layer, and immune cells. In between these cells are protein complexes called tight junctions that regulate what substance may pass between the cells. The GI microbiome the population of microbes with beneficial effects living in our gut also appears to play an important protective role.

Leaky gut is proposed to be caused by increased permeability of the GI lining. This may be due to injury to the mucosal surface, increased transport of substances across the inner lining, or disturbance of the microbiome. The resulting inflammation is considered to blame for multiple possible related conditions.

Various stressors are believed to contribute to leaky gut, including medical conditions, diet, and certain medications. Proposed risk factors for leaky gut syndrome include:

- Family history of gastrointestinal disorders such as inflammatory bowel disease or celiac disease
- A diet high in sugar, fat, and processed foods
- Infections, such as Helicobacter pylori (H. pylori)
- Alcohol
- Stress
- Diabetes

Certain medications like non-steroidal anti-inflammatory drugs (NSAIDs) and antibiotics

Unfortunately, there is no tried and true diagnostic test for leaky gut. Current tests involve consuming a "probe molecule," such as a large sugar molecule like lactulose, which the body doesn't normally absorb. The molecules are then measured in the urine to determine how much they've been absorbed. Unfortunately, there are no standards for this testing and normal results have not been determined.

Evaluation of gastrointestinal disease, in general, may include the following tests:

Laboratory studies, including a complete blood count (CBC) to look for anemia and signs of infection and a comprehensive metabolic panel to look for electrolyte abnormalities and to assess kidney and liver function.

Stool tests for ova and parasites, Clostridium dificile (C. diff) toxin, and white blood cells.

Imaging tests such as abdominal ultrasound or computed tomography (CT scan) to evaluate for gallbladder, liver, and pancreatic diseases.

Endoscopy, which is a test performed by a gastroenterologist (specialists who treat conditions of the GI system) that uses a probe to view the GI tract. An upper endoscopy can be used to evaluate the esophagus, stomach, and upper small intestine; and a colonoscopy is used to view the colon.

Treatments for Leaky Gut

Leaky gut is not a generally recognized clinical diagnosis at this time, and treatments to improve intestinal barrier function are under investigation.

Some treatments and dietary modifications have been proposed to affect the intestinal lining, however, more research is needed.

Proposed therapeutic strategies include:

- Stress avoidance
- Dietary changes, such as avoiding excess sugar, limiting fats, and increasing fiber
- Taking probiotics
- Taking supplements such as arginine or glutamine
- Consuming herbs, including ginger, peppermint, and tea
- Consuming certain mushrooms, broccoli, berries, and yogurt
- Avoiding certain medications such as NSAIDs
- Consuming a low FODMAP diet: FODMAPs are fermentable oligo-, di-, monosaccharides and

polyols, that are suggested to trigger symptoms. A low FODMAP diet limits wheat, dairy, legumes, and certain produce.

Prevention for Leaky Gut

While leaky gut is not a generally recognized clinical condition, there are some hypothetical ways to prevent impaired intestinal barrier. For example, we know that stress, infections, and some medications affect the gut lining. So you can consider the following to keep a healthy gut:

- Managing stress
- Avoiding NSAIDs
- Avoiding excess sugar and processed foods
- Limiting alcohol
- Taking a probiotic

- Practice proper hygiene when preparing foods to prevent GI illness

Related Conditions

Several conditions are proposed to have a link to leaky gut. A strong association has been found with intestinal disorders and certain other conditions. Studies have shown altered levels of various proteins and immune factors involved in the intestinal barrier in the following:

- Crohn's disease
- Celiac disease and gluten sensitivity
- Irritable bowel syndrome (IBS)
- Human immunodeficiency virus (HIV)
- Intestinal graft vs host disease (GVHD)

Proponents of leaky gut syndrome also suggest that the following conditions may be linked. However, studies are very limited or lacking evidence, and more research needs to be done before claiming that leaky gut syndrome causes them:

- Autoimmune conditions, such as autoimmune hepatitis, arthritis, type 1 diabetes, multiple sclerosis, and lupus
- Chronic fatigue syndrome
- Mood disorders like anxiety and depression
- Neurologic disorders such as Parkinson's disease and Alzheimer's disease

Your gut houses trillions of bacteria, collectively known as gut microbiota.

Several factors, including your diet, body weight, stress, and medication use, influence your gut bacteria. Good gut health, including a balanced gut environment and healthy gut lining, is essential for overall health as your gut impacts your entire body as well as your mood, sleep quality, and more.

If you have an unhealthy gut, it may lead to digestive issues such as diarrhea and chronic bloating, as well as other symptoms and health conditions. Fortunately, there are several ways to care for and improve your gut health, some of which don't have to do with your diet.

Here's everything you need to know about gut health and steps you can take to repair your gut.

How Do You Repair Your Gut Health?

Your gut contains an array of microorganisms. While some gut microorganisms are known to have anti-inflammatory effects, others can promote inflammation and harm gut health when their numbers get too high.

When your gut becomes imbalanced known as dysbiosis in the medical field there's a loss of beneficial microorganisms and an overgrowth of microorganisms that have the potential to harm health and create an inflammatory gut environment.

Several factors, some of which are out of your control, contribute to dysbiosis. For example, genetics and certain infections can alter the gut microbiota. However, factors within your control, such as diet and lifestyle, are among the most important contributors to gut dysbiosis.

Dysbiosis can negatively impact overall health and has been associated with a number of medical conditions, from gastrointestinal diseases to certain cancers.

Fortunately, no matter the cause of dysbiosis, there are several ways to improve the health of your gut and encourage a balanced microbial community within your gastrointestinal tract.

Increase Your Fiber Intake

A high-fiber diet has been shown to promote the health of beneficial bacteria in the gut and reduce the risk of several gut-related health conditions, such as colorectal cancer and diverticular disease.

Some fibrous foods, like artichokes and beans, are high in special fibers called prebiotics. Bacteria in your large intestine ferment prebiotics and release compounds called short-chain fatty acids (SCFAs). SCFAs provide energy for the cells that line your intestinal tract and are also involved in functions essential to gut health, such as mucus production and the regulation of intestinal pH.

Research shows that people who follow high-fiber diets have healthier guts, including increased microbial diversity, which is a sign of good gut health, compared to people who consume low amounts of dietary fiber.

Increasing your intake of high-fiber plant foods, such as vegetables, fruits, nuts, and beans, is an important part of caring for your gut and encouraging a balanced microbial community.

Cut Back on Added Sugar and Ultra-Processed Foods

A diet high in added sugar and ultra-processed foods can harm your gut barrier function and contribute to a pro-inflammatory gut environment.

For example, research shows that high added sugar and ultra-processed food intake can result in an unfavorable microbiota composition by decreasing the abundance of beneficial bacteria, such as Bacteroidetes species, while increasing the growth of Proteobacteria in the gut, which have pro-inflammatory properties.

Interestingly, the gut microbiota of people who consume high-sugar diets is similar to the microbiota of people with health conditions such as metabolic disorders and inflammatory bowel diseases (IBD). Cutting back on ultra-processed foods and foods and drinks high in added sugar and increasing your intake of nutritious foods is an easy way to heal your gut.

Avoid Unnecessary Medication Use

Although some medications are necessary, the overuse of certain medications, including antibiotics and proton pump inhibitors (PPIs), can negatively affect your gut.

Antibiotics harm your digestive health by releasing chemicals that disturb the gut microbiota, which can lead to the overgrowth of opportunistic microorganisms. Chronic antibiotic use has been linked to dysbiosis, so avoiding the unnecessary use of antibiotics is recommended.

PPIs can negatively impact gut health, too, especially with long-term use. PPIs reduce gastric acid secretion, which decreases microbial diversity and induces dysbiosis.

Maintain a Healthy Body Weight

Research indicates that obesity is associated with increased gut permeability, which is a sign of an unhealthy gut.

A healthy gut is lined with a tight barrier that controls what travels across the gut lining and into the bloodstream. When the gut lining becomes permeable, also known as "leaky gut", it allows material such as undigested food and toxins, to cross over into the bloodstream and other tissues, which contributes to low-grade inflammation.

What's more, people with obesity are more likely to have gut dysbiosis, though research suggests that dysbiosis can both contribute to obesity and be caused by obesity. People with obesity seem to have less bacterial diversity compared to people considered to be at a healthy weight.

Don't Smoke or Drink Excessively

Smoking cigarettes and drinking heavily can harm your health in a number of ways, including altering gut bacteria and contributing to dysbiosis. Smoking elevates intestinal pH, which promotes the growth of pathogenic bacteria while reducing the number of beneficial microorganisms. This may be part of the reason why smoking cigarettes is considered a major risk factor for digestive conditions such as Crohn's disease and peptic ulcers.

Chronic alcohol use is also associated with negative changes to the gut microbiota. People with alcohol use disorder have different gut microbiota compared to people who don't drink excessively. Alcohol abuse leads to dysbiosis and well as increased gut permeability, both of which can harm gut health.

For these reasons, cutting back on drinking and quitting smoking should be a priority if you're trying to heal your gut.

Studies show that diets high in certain foods are linked to a healthier gut. Incorporating the following foods into your diet may help improve gut health.

Fermented Foods

Fermented foods, such as kimchi, yogurt, kefir, and sauerkraut, are foods that are produced using controlled microbial growth. Fermentation helps preserve foods and improve taste and texture. The fermentation process produces beneficial bacteria, such as lactic acid bacteria (LAB), which are probiotic bacteria that positively impact human health.

According to study findings, diets rich in fermented foods may help protect against gut dysbiosis, encourage the growth of beneficial bacteria, and even improve symptoms of certain digestive conditions, such as IBS and IBD.

Fruits and Vegetables

Fruits and vegetables are rich in fiber as well as anti-inflammatory nutrients and phytochemicals, such as vitamin C, flavonols, phenolic acids, and anthocyanins, that can help encourage a healthy gut environment.

Diets high in fruits and vegetables have been shown to increase gut bacteria diversity and the number of beneficial bacteria such as Bifidobacterium and Lactobacillus, which are signs of a healthy gut.

Beans and Lentils

Beans and lentils are high in fiber and provide a type of fiber called resistant starch.

Resistant starch is fermented by gut bacteria, which leads to the production of short chain fatty acids (SCFAs), which promote gut health by fueling the cells that line your intestinal tract, regulating mucus production, and more.

Try adding lentils, chickpeas, black beans, and kidney beans to dishes like salads, grain bowls, and soups.

Nuts and seeds

Adding more nuts and seeds into your diet, like walnuts, flax seeds, and pecans, can help promote gut health in a number of ways. Studies show that diets rich in nuts and seeds may help encourage the growth of beneficial bacteria in your gut.

Plus, regularly eating fiber-rich nuts and seeds may help reduce your risk of certain digestive diseases like colon cancer.

Oats

Whole grains are a good source of soluble fiber. Oats contain a type of soluble fiber called beta glucan, which is fermented by bacteria in the large intestine. The fermentation process produces beneficial SCFAs, which promote digestive health and encourage a balanced gut.

Studies show that consuming oats may help stimulate SCFA production and promote the growth of beneficial bacteria like Bifidobacterium and Lactobacillus species in healthy people and in people with digestive conditions like celiac disease.

BreakFast

10-minute Blueberry Oatmeal

Ingredients

1 cup 2% or skim milk

1 cup gluten-free quick-cooking oats

1/4 cup raw honey

1/2 teaspoon ground cinnamon

½ teaspoon pure vanilla extract

3/4 cup fresh or frozen unsweetened blueberries, thawed

1 tablespoon sliced almonds

Directions

Place a saucepan in medium heat. Add milk and bring to a boil. Stir in the oats and cook for 2 minutes, or until thick; stirring occasionally. Add the honey, cinnamon, and vanilla and blend well. Ladle oatmeal into bowls and top with blueberries.

Ingredients

4 organic free-range eggs, beaten

1 tomato, seeded and chopped

1 pinch salt and pepper, or to taste

1/4 cup gluten-free Cheddar cheese, grated

1/2 cup broccoli florets, chopped

1 medium red bell pepper, diced

1 medium onion, chopped

2 cloves garlic, crushed and chopped

1 tablespoon olive oil

Directions

Heat olive oil in a skillet over medium-high heat. Add garlic and onion and sauté until garlic is lightly browned and onion is soft.

Stir in broccoli and cook for about 5 minutes, or until tender. Turn heat to medium. Add the beaten eggs and cook for 2 minutes.

Mix in the tomato and red bell pepper. Season with salt and pepper. Stir occasionally and cook until eggs are set. Serve warm with sprinkled cheese on top.

Blueberry Buckwheat Pancakes

Ingredients

1 teaspoon coconut oil

1 3/4 cup organic coconut butter (recommended: Artisana)

1 1/2 cup buckwheat flour

1/8 teaspoon salt

3 tablespoon raw honey

1 teaspoon baking soda

2 tablespoon pure maple syrup

1/4 cup frozen blueberries

Directions

Combine the buckwheat flour, salt, honey, and baking soda in a large mixing bowl.

Whisk together the egg and 1 1/2 cup coconut butter. Add egg mixture to the buckwheat batter gently. Let the batter stand for 10 minutes (or overnight). Place a saucepan over medium heat. Add 1 teaspoon of coconut butter and melt. Ladle 1/4 cup of batter onto the pan to for each pancake. Turn the pancakes over once bubbles burst on top; cook the other side until golden brown. Place pancakes in serving plates and top with 1 teaspoon each of the remaining butter and frozen blueberries.

Gluten Free Banana Bread

Ingredients

1 cup white rice

1/2 cup ground oats

1/4 cup almond meal

1/4 cup flax meal

1 teaspoon baking powder

1/2 teaspoon sea salt

1/2 cup coconut oil, melted, and 1 tablespoon for greasing

1/4 cup raw honey

6 ripe bananas, mashed

2 organic free-range eggs, lightly beaten

3 tablespoons maple syrup

1 teaspoon cinnamon

1 pinch nutmeg

Directions

Preheat oven to 350 degrees F. Grease a 9x5 inch loaf pan lightly with 1 tablespoon coconut oil. Mix together the white rice, ground oats, almond meal, flax meal, baking powder and salt in a large mixing bowl. In another large bowl, stir together the eggs, coconut oil, honey, maple syrup, cinnamon, nutmeg, and bananas. Add the flour mixture and mix well to produce a moist batter. Transfer batter to the loaf pan. Bake for 20-30 minutes, or until a toothpick inserted into center of the loaf comes out clean or with only a few crumbs sticking to it. If using muffin or cupcake tins, bake for 15 minutes, or until a toothpick inserted into the center of a muffin comes out clean.

Gluten Free Almond-Raspberry Danish Tartlets

Ingredients

Crust and Filling:

2 cups gluten-free pancake mix

1/4 cup almond butter, room temperature

2 tablespoons Stevia

2/3 cup almond milk

1/2 teaspoon almond extract

1/4 cup organic raspberry jam

Glaze and Garnish:

2/3 cup Stevia

2 tablespoons milk, or more as needed

1/2 teaspoon pure vanilla extract

1/4 teaspoon almond extract

1/2 cup chopped almonds

Directions

Preheat an oven to 400 degrees F (200 degrees C). Line a baking sheet with parchment paper.

Make the crusts: In a large mixing bowl, mix together the pancake mix, butter, and 2 tablespoons Stevia until crumbly. Stir in 2/3 cup milk and 1/2 teaspoon almond extract; mix well to incorporate. Drop several tablespoonful of dough onto the baking sheet; place each dough ball 2 inches apart. Make a hollow on each dough ball by pressing the back of a teaspoon in the center. Fill each center with 1 teaspoon of raspberry jam. Bake for 10-12 minutes, or until lightly browned.

Make the glaze: Stir together all the glaze ingredients (except for the chopped almonds) until smooth. Drizzle the glaze over the tartlets and sprinkle chopped almonds over the top.

Breakfast Gluten-free Brownies

Ingredients

1 1/2 cups gluten-free quick-cooking oats

3/4 cup carob powder

1/2 cup gluten-free all-purpose baking flour

1 teaspoon baking powder

3/4 cup raw honey

3/4 cup flax seed meal

1/2 teaspoon ground cinnamon

1/4 teaspoon salt

1/4 cup rice milk

1 teaspoon pure vanilla extract

1 organic free-range egg

1 ripe banana, mashed

1 tablespoon coconut oil for greasing

Directions

Preheat oven to 350 degrees F (175 degrees C). Lightly grease an 8x10-inch baking pan.

In a large mixing bowl, combine the first 8 ingredients. In another mixing bowl, stir together the rice milk, vanilla, and banana. Stir in the banana mixture into flour mixture. Transfer batter into the prepared baking pan.

Bake for about 20 minutes, or until a toothpick inserted in the center comes out clean. Cover pan and allow brownies to cool for at least 5 minutes. Slice into bars and serve.

Spinach and Berries Smoothie

Ingredients

1/2 cup frozen strawberries

1/2 cup frozen blueberries

1 cup fresh spinach leaves, chopped

1 ripe banana, peeled and chopped

1/2 cup soy milk

1/2 cup fat-free plain yogurt

1 1/2 tablespoons flax seeds

1 teaspoon honey

Directions

Combine all ingredients in a blender and blend until smooth. Pour into glasses and serve.

Quick Scrambled Egg N' Mushrooms

Ingredients

1/4 cup olive oil

3 cloves garlic, crushed and chopped

1/4 cup onions, chopped

1/4 cup green bell peppers, chopped

1/4 cup fresh mushrooms, sliced

6 eggs, beaten

1/4 cup fresh tomato, chopped

salt and freshly ground black pepper, to taste

Directions

Place a skillet over medium-high heat. Add the olive oil. Once oil is hot, add the garlic and sauté until lightly browned.

Stir in the mushrooms, onions, bell peppers, and tomatoes and cook until onions are soft. Stir in the beaten eggs and cook for 1 minute, or until egg is set. Slice into wedges and serve.

Gluten-free Sugar-free Granola

Ingredients

5 cups gluten-free rolled oats

2 cups unsalted almonds, chopped

1 cup unsalted hazelnuts, chopped

3/4 cup sesame seeds

2 teaspoons ground cinnamon

1 teaspoon ground nutmeg

1 teaspoon sea salt

1/2 cup dried dates

1/2 cup dried prunes

1/2 cup dried cranberries

3/4 cup agave syrup (or raw honey)

1 tablespoon pure vanilla extract

2 tablespoons coconut oil

Directions

Preheat the oven to 350°.

In a large roasting pan, combine the oats, almonds, hazelnuts, and sesame seeds, and then stir in the cinnamon, nutmeg, and salt. Add the dried fruits and toss well. Drizzle mixture with maple syrup, vanilla, and coconut oil, and toss to coat.

Bake for 12 minutes. Stir with a fork once halfway through. Let cool and serve.

Ingredients

Crust:

1/4 cup raw walnuts, chopped

1 cup dates, pitted

1/4 cup carob powder

1/2 teaspoon pure vanilla extract

2 teaspoon water, 1 pinch salt

Mousse:

3/4 cup avocado, chopped

1/4 cup carob powder

1 ripe banana

2 tablespoons agave syrup

1/2 teaspoon pure vanilla extract

Directions

Place all ingredients for the crust in a blender or food
processor and process until a dough consistency is

reached. Using your hands, press down the dough in a shallow dish. Process all mousse ingredients in a blender or food processor until creamy. Pour mousse over the crust. Place cake in the refrigerator to chill.

Summer Fresh Fruit Salad

Ingredients

6 bananas, peeled and sliced

2 cups strawberries, hulled and halved

2 cups cantaloupe balls

1/2 cup seedless green grapes

2 ripe bananas, sliced

1/2 cup blackberries or blueberries

Dressing:

1/2 cup nonfat lemon yogurt

1/4 cup raw honey

1/2 cup fresh lemon juice

5 sprigs fresh mint, chopped

Directions

Place fruits in a large bowl.

Combine dressing ingredients in a small bowl and pour

over fruits. Gently toss to coat.

Cover and refrigerate before serving.

Avocado Omelet

Ingredients

2 cloves garlic, crushed and chopped

1/2 cup mushroom, diced

1 large tomato, diced

1 medium onion, chopped

3 cups baby spinach leaves, chopped

1 avocado flesh, mashed

8 eggs

salt and pepper to taste

2 tablespoons olive oil

Directions

Heat olive oil in a skillet over medium heat. Add the garlic and sauté until lightly browned.

Stir in the mushroom, tomato, onion, spinach, and mashed avocado; season with a pinch of salt and pepper. Cook vegetables until tender. In a medium bowl, beat the eggs and season with salt and pepper. Pour the egg mixture in the skillet and cook for 3 minutes on each side, or until set.

Flax-Almond Porridge

Ingredients

2 bananas, mashed

2 cups almond milk

1 teaspoon raw honey

3/4 cup almond meal

1/4 cup flax meal

1 teaspoon ground cinnamon

1/4 cup organic pure maple syrup

1 apple, diced

Directions

Place a saucepan over medium heat. Add and stir together almond meal, flax meal, almond milk, honey, and bananas until smooth. Sprinkle cinnamon over mixture.

Simmer for about 3-4 minutes, or until thick and bubbly.

Pour porridge into bowls. Add diced apples on top and drizzle with maple syrup.

Banana and Blueberry French Toast

Ingredients

1 tablespoon coconut oil (for greasing)

1 loaf gluten-free sliced bread

4 organic free-range eggs

1 teaspoon cinnamon

1 dash salt

1/4 cup coconut milk or almond milk

1/2 cup organic pure maple syrup

1/2 cup frozen blueberries

1/2 cup sliced ripe bananas

Directions

Preheat a skillet to 350 degrees F.

Beat together eggs, cinnamon, sea salt, and coconut milk in a medium bowl. Grease a skillet with coconut oil and place over medium heat.

Coat each bread slice with the egg mixture and cook each side in the skillet for 3-4 minutes.

Place toasts in serving plates and top with blueberries and bananas, then drizzle maple syrup over the top.

Pan Fried Halibut with Cilantro Tartar Sauce

Ingredients

Fish fillet:

4 halibut fillets, skinless (or any white fish)

2 eggs

1 1/2 cups coconut flour

1 tablespoon garam masala

1 teaspoon salt

1/2 teaspoon freshly ground black pepper

1 teaspoon garlic powder

1/4 cup olive oil

Cilantro Tartar Sauce:

2 tablespoons fresh cilantro

1 cup gluten-free mayonnaise

1/4 cup onion, finely chopped

1 tablespoon lemon juice

1/2 teaspoon dried dill

Directions

Stir together all tartar sauce ingredients and chill for 30 minutes.

Beat the eggs in a bowl. In a separate bowl, stir together the coconut flour, garam masala, salt, garlic powder, and pepper. Coat each side of the fish fillet in the egg mixture, and then in the flour mixture.

Place a skillet over medium heat. Add the olive oil. When oil is hot, cook coated fillets on each side for 5 minutes, or until golden brown. Place fish fillets in plates. Serve with tartar sauce and steamed veggies.

Gluten-Free Cream of Mushroom Soup

Ingredients

8 ounces fresh mushrooms, sliced

1/4 cup shallots, chopped

1/2 cup cauliflower florets

1 tablespoon fresh thyme, chopped, 1 bay leaf

2 cloves garlic, minced, 3 tablespoons olive oil

4 tablespoons gluten-free corn flour dissolved in 4 tablespoons water

1 cup low-sodium chicken stock

1 cup light cream

1/2 teaspoon salt

1/4 teaspoon freshly ground black pepper

Directions

Heat olive oil in a 3 quart saucepan over medium heat. Add garlic and sauté until brown. Stir in the mushrooms, cauliflower, and shallots and cook for about 3 minutes.

Pour in dissolved corn flour and stir, about 2 minutes.

Slowly pour the chicken stock. Add the thyme, bay leaf, and light cream; blend well until thick. Season with salt and pepper to taste.

Ladle soup into bowls and serve.

Hot Summer Chili

Ingredients

2 tablespoons extra-virgin olive oil

2 large red onion, chopped

5 cloves garlic, crushed

2 tablespoons ground cayenne pepper

2 cups fresh tomatoes, chopped

1 cup black beans, drained

1 cup light kidney beans, drained

1 cup low-sodium chicken broth

1/2 cup green bell pepper, chopped

1/2 cup red bell pepper, chopped

1 cup corn kernels

Salt and freshly ground black pepper, to taste

1/2 cup fresh cilantro, chopped

Directions

Sauté onion, garlic, and cayenne in a pot over medium heat for 5 minutes, or until onion is soft. Stir in all the other ingredients, except for the cilantro, and bring to a boil. Reduce heat to low and simmer for 20 minutes or until vegetables are soft. Serve topped with chopped fresh cilantro.

Salmon Egg Salad

Ingredients

14 ounces flaked salmon

1 medium red radish, diced

6 hard-boiled eggs, peeled and chopped

2 teaspoons chopped dill

1 1/2 teaspoons Dijon mustard

1/2-3/4 cup gluten-free mayonnaise

1/2 cup onion, chopped

1/2 teaspoon dried rosemary

1/2 sea salt

1/8 teaspoon black pepper

1/4 cup chives, chopped

Directions

Combine all ingredients in a large bowl; gently toss to coat. Chill for at least an hour and serve.

Fruity Chicken Salad

Ingredients

1 1/2 pounds boneless chicken breast halves - cooked, cooled and cubed

1 cup oranges, drained

1 cup pineapple chunks, drained

2 cup gluten-free macaroni (cooked according to package instructions)

1/2 cup almonds, sliced

1 cup gluten-free light mayonnaise

2 teaspoons dried dill weed

2 teaspoons honey

Directions

Stir together the mayonnaise, dill weed, and honey in a small bowl. Combine the chicken, macaroni, oranges, pineapple and almonds in a large mixing bowl. Pour dressing over chicken-fruit mixture and toss to coat. Chill in the fridge for at least 1 hour before serving.

BLT Salad

Ingredients

1 pound gluten-free bacon (recommended: Augason Farms, Hormel Foods, Range Brand)

3/4 cup gluten-free mayonnaise

1/4 cup low-fat milk

1 teaspoon garlic powder

1/8 teaspoon ground black pepper

¼ teaspoon salt, 1 head romaine lettuce, shredded

2 large tomatoes, chopped

1 cup almonds, sliced

Directions

Drizzle skillet with olive oil and heat over medium high. Add bacon and cook until browned and crisp. Drain on paper towels. Crumble and set aside. Stir together mayonnaise, milk, garlic powder, salt and black pepper in a small bowl until smooth. In a large salad bowl, mix together the lettuce, tomatoes, bacon, and almonds. Pour dressing over bacon mixture. Toss well and serve.

Cedar Planked Salmon Fillets

Ingredients

2 (2 pound) salmon fillets, skin removed

1/3 cup gluten-free soy sauce

1/3 cup olive oil

1 1/2 tablespoons rice vinegar

1/4 cup green onions, chopped

1 teaspoon garlic, minced

1 tablespoon fresh ginger, grated

1 cup fresh dill, chopped

½ cup onions, chopped

1 fresh lemon, juiced

Directions

Soak 3 (12-inch) untreated cedar planks in warm water for at least 1 hour, but overnight would be even better. Place the salmon fillets in a shallow dish. Mix together the soy sauce, olive oil, green onions, rice vinegar, garlic, and ginger in a small bowl. Rub the marinade into salmon fillets. Cover and marinate for 15-60 minutes. In a medium bowl, combine dill, onions and lemon juice. Press mixture onto the top side of the fillets.

Preheat an outdoor grill for medium heat. Place the planks on the grill with the lid closed, for 3 minutes, or until they start to crackle and smoke. Place the fillets carefully onto the planks, skin side down; spacing fillets 1 inch apart. Cover, and grill for about 20 minutes. Remove planks from the grill. Place fillets onto plates and serve.

Chicken Fruit Spinach Salad

Ingredients

1 1/2 cups cooked chicken, cut into bite-size pieces

8 ounces fresh spinach, torn into bite-size pieces

2 cups strawberries, hulled and sliced

2 cups mandarin orange segments

1/4 cup toasted walnuts, sliced

Dressing:

3 tablespoons sesame seeds

1/2 cup raw honey

1/2 cup olive oil

1/4 cup balsamic vinegar

1/4 teaspoon gluten-free Worcestershire sauce

1 medium onion, minced

1/2 tablespoon Dijon mustard

salt and pepper, to taste

Directions

Whisk together all the dressing ingredients in a bowl. Cover and chill for one hour. In a large bowl, combine the chicken, spinach, strawberries, orange, and walnuts. Pour dressing over salad. Toss ingredients well to coat. Chill for 15 minutes then serve.

Thai Chicken Noodle Soup

Ingredients

6 cups low-sodium chicken broth

1-2 fresh chicken breasts , chopped

1 stalk lemongrass, minced

1 bay leaf

1 tablespoon ginger, grated

1 large carrot, sliced

1 cup broccoli florets, trimmed

1 cup mushrooms, quartered

1/2 teaspoon. cayenne pepper

3 cloves garlic, minced

1/4 cup fresh lime juice

2 Tablespoon. gluten free soy sauce

1/4 cup coconut milk

Salt and black pepper (to taste)

a handful fresh cilantro, chopped

8-10 oz. gluten-free flat Thai rice noodles

Directions

Boil noodles according to package directions, or until al dente. Drain and set aside. Pour chicken broth in a large pot and bring to a boil over high heat. Add chicken, broccoli, mushrooms, lemongrass, ginger, carrot, bay leaf. Turn heat to high and allow broth to boil for 1 minute. Cover the pot and reduce heat to medium. Simmer soup for 6 more minutes. While soup is simmering, stir in cayenne, garlic, lime juice, and soy sauce. Turn heat to low and add the coconut milk; stir well. Place cooked noodles into bowls. Pour soup over the noodles, then sprinkle with cilantro.

Gluten-Free Pepperoni Pizza

Ingredients

1 (12-inch) Gluten Free refrigerated pizza crust dough (recommended: Bob's Red Mill, Pillsbury,)

¾ cup gluten-free pizza sauce

1 cup part-skim mozzarella cheese, shredded

30 slices gluten-free turkey pepperoni slices

2 medium tomatoes, diced

1/2 cup onion, chopped

Directions

Preheat oven to 400°F.

Press dough into a greased baking sheet. Bake for 8 minutes. Remove dough from oven. Spread pizza sauce over dough. Add remaining ingredients on top. Return pizza into oven and bake for 6 to 9 minutes longer or until crusts are deep golden brown and cheese is melted. Divide into wedges and serve.

Quick N' Easy Gluten Free Chicken Stir Fry

Ingredients

1 tablespoon olive oil

1 1/2 pound boneless chicken breast cut into 1 inch cubes

2 cloves garlic, minced

1 small onion, chopped

1 cup mushrooms, sliced

2 cups broccoli, chopped

1 medium carrot, sliced

1/2 cup low-sodium chicken broth

3 tablespoon coconut aminos

1 teaspoon raw honey

1 teaspoon corn flour dissolved in 1 teaspoon water

1/4 teaspoon ground black pepper

Directions

Heat olive oil in a skillet over medium heat. Add the chicken, garlic, and onions; cook for 5 minutes or until chicken is golden brown. Stir in the mushrooms and cook for 10 minutes more. Add broccoli, carrots, chicken broth and coconut aminos, and pepper. Cover and simmer for 5 more minutes. Stir in corn flour and simmer until sauce thickens.

Easy Baked Tilapia

Ingredients

1 pound tilapia fillets, about 4 fillets

3 tablespoons organic butter, melted

1 tablespoon olive oil

1 tablespoon fresh lemon juice

2 cloves garlic, minced

1 teaspoon Stevia

1/2 teaspoon pepper

1/2 teaspoon dried thyme

1 tablespoon parsley, chopped

1/3 cup gluten-free breadcrumbs

1 lemon, sliced

Directions

Preheat oven to 425. Grease a 9x13 inch baking dish lightly with olive oil.

Rinse fish filets and pat dry. Layer fillets in the prepared baking dish.

Stir together the garlic, butter, lemon juice, Stevia, thyme, parsley, and pepper in a small bowl. Pour and rub mixture over fish fillets; marinate for at least 15 minutes.

Sprinkle fillets with the breadcrumbs.

Bake for about 20 minutes or until fillets are flakey. Garnish with lemon slices.

Gluten-Free, Dairy-Free Cherry Turkey Lettuce Wraps

Ingredients

4 tablespoons olive oil

1 1/2 cup yellow onion, diced

1 tablespoon garlic, minced

1 tablespoon ginger, minced

1 pound ground turkey

1/2 cup toasted almonds, sliced

1/2 cup fresh cilantro, chopped

2 tablespoons coconut aminos

1 teaspoon raw honey

1 teaspoon salt

1 teaspoon freshly ground black pepper

8 large iceberg lettuce leaves

1/2 cup dark sweet cherries, pitted and halved

Directions

Heat olive oil in a skillet over medium-high heat. Add the onions and garlic and sauté for about 5 minutes until lightly browned.

Stir in the turkey and cook for 8-10 minutes until the meat is no longer pink inside.

Add the almonds, cilantro, coconut aminos, and honey and cook for 3 minutes. Season with the salt and pepper.

Fill each lettuce leaf with a heaping spoonful of meat mixture and cherries.

Gluten Free Chicken Piccata

Ingredients

4 boneless, skinless, organic, free-range chicken breast halves, pounded

1 cup ground almond meal

1/4 cup grated Parmesan cheese

1/2 teaspoon Dijon mustard

1 yellow onion, chopped

1 teaspoon sea salt

1/2 teaspoon freshly ground black pepper

4 tablespoons olive oil

4 tablespoons organic unsalted butter

1/2 cup organic gluten-free chicken broth

3 tablespoons lemon juice, freshly squeezed

2 tablespoons capers, rinsed

3 tablespoons organic butter

1/4 cup fresh parsley, chopped

Directions

Combine the almond meal, cheese, mustard, salt, and pepper together spread the mixture on a shallow dish. Rinse the pounded chicken breasts in water and shake off the excess. Dredge the chicken in the flour mixture. Melt 2 tablespoons butter in a large skillet over medium high heat; add the olive oil.

Cook chicken in butter and oil for approximately 3-4 minutes on each side until golden brown.

Place cooked chicken breasts on a serving dish and cover to keep warm.

Stir in the chicken broth, lemon juice and capers, scraping up any brown bits in the pan.

Add the chicken broth, lemon juice, and capers to the skillet; stirring and scraping up any brown bits in the skillet. Simmer until the sauce is reduced and reaches a light syrup consistency. Reduce heat to low and stir in remaining butter.

Spoon the sauce over the chicken breasts, top with chopped parsley. Serve with lemon slices or wedges.

Pork Tenderloin in Cranberry-Spinach Salad

Ingredients

1 pound pork tenderloin

1 cup cider vinegar

1 teaspoon Dijon mustard

1/4 cup raw honey

1 teaspoon dried thyme, crushed

3 tablespoons toasted sesame seeds

2 tablespoon raw honey

2 medium shallots, sliced

2 cloves garlic, crushed and chopped

1 cup dried cranberries

3/4 cup toasted pine nuts

1 pound baby spinach leaves, rinsed and torn into bite-size pieces

Directions

Preheat oven to 425 degrees F.

Place meat in shallow pan. Mix together cider vinegar, mustard, 1/4 cup honey and thyme in a bowl and brush the sauce mixture onto meat. Bake meat for 20-25 minutes. Slice meat into bite-size pieces and place into a large bowl.

Whisk together the sesame seeds, 2 tablespoons honey, shallots, garlic, 1/2 cup cider vinegar and olive oil and pour onto the meat. Add spinach, pine nuts and cranberries; toss well and serve.

Dijonnaise Tuna Salad on a Bed of Lettuce

Ingredients

1 (6 ounce) oil-packed tuna

1/2 cup gluten-free mayonnaise

1/4 cup walnuts, chopped

1 medium ripe avocado, sliced into chunks

1/4 cup scallions, minced

1 tablespoon Dijon mustard

1 medium onion, chopped

1 apple, cored and diced

4 leaves lettuce

Sea salt and pepper to taste

1 teaspoon sweet pickle relish

Directions

Whisk together the mayonnaise, mustard, salt, and pepper in a medium bowl. Toss in tuna, onion, apple, walnuts, scallions and pickle relish. Cover and chill for 10 minutes.

Line the lettuce leaves on serving plates and fill the center with tuna mixture, then add avocado chunks on top.

Gluten free Teriyaki Salmon

Ingredients

4 (6 ounce) salmon steaks

Sauce:

1/4 cup gluten-free soy sauce (or coconut aminos)

1 teaspoon olive oil

1/2 cup lemon juice

1 tablespoon honey

1 tablespoon ginger, minced

1 teaspoon garlic, minced

1/2 cup spring onions, finely chopped

1/4 teaspoon ground black pepper

1 stalk lemongrass, minced

1 tablespoon sesame seeds

Directions

Preheat the oven to 180°C. Line a baking sheet with grease-proof or wax paper. In a small bowl, whisk together the sauce ingredients. Place the salmon into a large dish and pour the prepared sauce over the salmon and refrigerate for at least 30 minutes. Transfer the salmon to the baking sheet and bake for 10-12 minutes or until cooked through. Serve with your choice of vegetable salad.

Honey Mustard Grilled Pork Chops

Ingredients

8 thin cut pork chops

1/3 cup raw honey

3 tablespoons lemon juice

1 teaspoon Frank's Red hot sauce

1 tablespoon apple cider vinegar

1 teaspoon gluten free Worcestershire sauce

2 teaspoons onion powder

1/4 teaspoon dried rosemary

3 tablespoons Dijon mustard

1 teaspoon cranberry juice

Directions

Place honey, lemon juice, hot sauce vinegar, cranberry juice, Worcestershire sauce, onion powder, rosemary, and mustard in a large re-sealable plastic bag.

Place pork chops in the plastic bag, tightly seal and gently shake to coat. Place bag in the refrigerator for at least 2 hours to marinate. Discard marinade and grill pork chops over high heat for 6-8 minutes.

Beef Stuffed Cabbage

Ingredients

1 medium head cabbage

1 pound ground beef

1 cup cooked gluten free brown rice

1 organic, free-range egg

1 tablespoon dried parsley flakes

1/2 teaspoon garlic powder

2 celery stalks with leaves, finely chopped

water to cover

1 1/2 cup gluten-free tomato sauce

1 tablespoon apple cider vinegar

1 tablespoon raw honey

Directions

In a large pot over high heat, add 2 quarts water and cabbage and bring to a boil for 15 minutes, or until outer leaves are tender. Drain cabbage and allow to cool completely. Using a paring knife, remove outer core of cabbage.

Mix together the beef, rice, egg, parsley flakes, garlic powder, and celery in a large bowl.

Fill the center of each cabbage leaf with 1/3 cup of the beef mixture. Fold sides over filling, tucking in the sides of the leaf.

Pile up the stuffed cabbage leaves in a large pot over medium low heat, placing the larger leaves on the bottom. Add the tomato sauce, vinegar, honey and enough water to cover. Simmer for about an hour, or until cabbage is very tender. Add tomato sauce as needed.

Raw Veggie Nuts and Seeds Salad

Ingredients

3 medium carrots, diced

1/2 cup radish, diced

1 medium cucumber, diced

3 celery ribs,

1 head cauliflower

1 green bell pepper

1 red bell pepper

1 cup green cabbage

1 small onion

1/4 cup fresh basil

salt and pepper

1/2 cup cashews, chopped

1/2 cup almonds, chopped

1/2 cup raw pumpkin seeds

1/2 cup raw sunflower seeds

1/2 tablespoon sea salt (or to taste)

Directions

Toss together all the vegetables in a large bowl.

Heat a skillet over medium heat. Dry roast the nuts and seeds until lightly browned and crisp. Season with salt and stir. Let cool, and then toss the roasted nuts and seeds with the vegetables. Serve with your choice of gluten-free salad dressing.

Parmigiano Beef Meatballs

Ingredients

1.5 pounds lean ground beef

3/4 cup gluten-free Parmigiano Reggiano, grated

1/2 cup flax meal

2 eggs

1/4 teaspoon garlic powder

1 medium onion, finely chopped

1 teaspoon sea salt

1/4 teaspoon freshly ground black pepper

1/2 cup warm water

1 cup gluten-free organic tomato sauce

Directions

Preheat oven to 350 degrees F. Mix all meatball ingredients in a large bowl and shape into 2-inch meatballs. Arrange meatballs on a baking sheet, about 1 1/2-inches apart. Bake for 20 minutes, or until internal temp reaches 160 degrees. Serve warm.

Grilled Rosemary Lime Swordfish

Ingredients

4 (4 ounce) swordfish steaks

2 teaspoons fresh rosemary, chopped (or 1 teaspoon dried rosemary)

3 cloves garlic, minced

1/2 cup white wine (or red wine vinegar)

1/4 teaspoon salt

1/4 teaspoon ground black pepper

2 tablespoon thinly sliced scallions

2 tablespoons lime juice

1 tablespoon finely chopped parsley

1 tablespoon olive oil

1 teaspoon dried thyme

4 slices lemon, for garnish

Directions

Place fish in a baking dish and season with salt and pepper. Combine garlic, 1 teaspoon rosemary, and white wine in a small bowl. Pour mixture over fish, turning to coat.

Cover, and place in fridge for at least 1 hour.

In a small bowl, stir together the scallions, lime juice, parsley, olive oil, thyme, and remaining rosemary.

Preheat grill for medium heat.

Grill fish for 10 minutes, turning once, or until fish is flakey. Place fish onto plates and pour the prepared lime sauce on top. Serve immediately.

Ingredients

2 pounds lean ground beef

1/2 cup gluten free teriyaki sauce

1 can (8 ounces) gluten free organic pineapple slices, juice reserved

4 lettuce leaves

4 slices Swiss cheese

4 slices tomato

4 gluten-free burger buns

Directions

Mix together beef and teriyaki sauce in a large bowl; season with salt and pepper.

Divide and form mixture into 4 patties, then drizzle each patty with the reserved pineapple juice. Place a pineapple slice on top of each patty.

Discard excess marinade. Grill the burgers over medium-low heat until cooked through.

Layer the burgers in the following order: top bun, lettuce, pineapple, cheese, burger patty, bottom bun.

Spinach N' Mushroom Stuffed Chicken

Ingredients

4 butterflied chicken breasts

1 cup button mushrooms, chopped

5 slices of nitrite and nitrate- free bacon

4-5 cups fresh spinach, chopped

1/2 teaspoon ground nutmeg

1 small onion, quartered

2 cloves garlic, minced

Salt, to taste

freshly ground black pepper, to taste

Toothpicks

Directions

Preheat oven to 350 degrees F. Line a baking sheet with parchment paper.

Place a large skillet over medium-high heat. Add the bacon slices and cook each side until crispy. Place cooked bacon in a plate lined with paper towel and let cool.

Cook bacon in a large skillet over medium-high heat until crispy. Drain in paper towels and let cool.

Leave about 3 tablespoons of excess bacon fat in the pan and discard the rest.

Add mushrooms and garlic and sauté until vegetables are softened and lightly browned. Season with salt and pepper. Stir in the spinach, sprinkle with ground nutmeg. Cover the skillet and allow vegetables to simmer until the spinach has wilted. Add the cooked bacon and mix well. Remove the pan from heat. Spoon mixture into chicken breasts and secure with toothpicks.

Place stuffed chicken breasts on the prepared baking sheet. Bake for 18-20 minutes, or until chicken is no longer pink in the center.

Grilled Tilapia with Black Bean Mango Salsa

Ingredients

2 (6 ounce) tilapia fillets

1 clove garlic, minced

1 tablespoon dried parsley flakes

1 teaspoon dried basil

1 tablespoon lemon juice

1/3 cup extra-virgin olive oil

1 teaspoon ground black pepper

1/2 teaspoon salt

Salsa:

1/2 cup black beans, rinsed and drained

1 large ripe mango, peeled, pitted and diced

1 tablespoon freshly squeezed orange juice

2 tablespoons lemon juice, freshly squeezed

2 tablespoons red onion, minced

1/2 red bell pepper, diced

1 tablespoon fresh cilantro, chopped

1 teaspoon ground cumin

1/4 teaspoon sea salt, or to taste

1/4 teaspoon ground black pepper, or to taste

Directions

In a mixing bowl, mix all the salsa ingredients and refrigerate until serving.

Place tilapia fillets in a large dish.

Whisk together the garlic, parsley, basil, lemon juice, olive oil, salt, and pepper in a bowl. Pour marinade onto fillets and turn sides to coat. Place in the fridge for 1 hour.

Preheat a lightly oiled grill to medium-high.

Discard tilapia marinade and grill the fillets 3-4 minutes each side, or until flesh is opaque in the center, and flakes easily with a fork. Serve the tilapia with mango salsa.

Grilled Lemon N' Lime Cod Fillets

Ingredients

1 pound cod, cut into 4 fillets (or other white fish)

Marinade:

2 tablespoons olive oil

1/4 cup fresh cilantro, chopped

1/2 teaspoon Stevia (or raw honey)

1 teaspoon sea salt

1/2 teaspoon black pepper

1/2 teaspoon cayenne pepper

1 tablespoon fresh lemon juice

1 tablespoon fresh lime juice

1 tablespoon lemon zest

1 tablespoon lime zest

Directions

Place fish in a large dish. Mix all ingredients for the marinade in a small bowl and pour over fish. Place in the fridge and marinate for 10-20 minutes.

Preheat a lightly oiled grill to medium-high.

Grill cod fillets for 4-6 minutes on each side, until golden brown.

Gluten-free Beef and Broccoli Stir-fry

Ingredients

Beef and Marinade:

1 pound beef flank steak, cut into strips

1/4 cup water

1/4 cup gluten-free soy sauce (or coconut aminos)

2 cloves garlic, minced

1/4 teaspoon ground pepper

Stir-Fry:

2 tablespoon olive oil

4 cups broccoli florets

1/2 cup onion, chopped

1/2 cup carrots, julienned

Sauce:

1 cup cold water

1/4 cup gluten-free soy sauce (or coconut aminos)

1/4 cup brown sugar

1 1/2 teaspoon ground ginger

1 teaspoon sesame oil

1/4 teaspoon red pepper flakes

1/4 cup cornstarch

Directions

In a large bowl, whisk together all the marinade ingredients. Add beef and marinate for 30 minutes.

Heat olive oil in a large pan or wok over medium-high heat. Stir in the beef and marinade, and cook for 3-5 minutes, or until meat is no longer pink.

Add onion and carrots, and fry for 2 minutes more; stirring often. Stir in the broccoli and fry for 1 more minute.

Whisk together all the sauce ingredients in a small bowl. Pour mixture over the beef and vegetable mixture, and cook for about 2-3 more minutes, or until sauce thickens. Serve over hot brown rice.

Lemon and Herb Crusted Salmon Fillets

Ingredients

4 (4-ounce) Atlantic Salmon Portions

2 teaspoons salt

1 teaspoon freshly ground black pepper

1 cup gluten-free breadcrumbs

2 tablespoons chives, finely chopped

2 tablespoons fresh thyme, finely chopped

2 tablespoons parsley, finely chopped

1 teaspoon Dijon mustard

1 teaspoon ginger, grated

1/2 teaspoon garlic powder

1/2 teaspoon onion powder

1 teaspoon lemon peel, grated

1/4 cup lemon juice

Directions

Preheat oven to 400 degrees F. Line a baking sheet with parchment paper.

Season both sides of salmon fillets with salt and pepper. Place skin side down on the prepared baking sheet.

Combine the breadcrumbs, chives, thyme, parsley, mustard, ginger, garlic powder, onion powder, and lemon peel in a medium bowl.

Sprinkle salmon with lemon juice and press the breadcrumb mixture on top of the salmon fillets.

Cook for 10- 15 minutes, or until cooked through.

Ingredients

Fish sticks:

1 pound white fish, cut into 1x5-inch pieces

2 organic free-range eggs, whisked

1/2 cup blanched almond flour

1/2 teaspoon ground cayenne pepper

1/4 cup dried basil

3 cloves garlic, finely chopped

1 teaspoon salt

1/4 teaspoon freshly ground black pepper

1/2 cup coconut oil

Garlic Lime Tartar Sauce:

1 cup mayonnaise

1 teaspoon garlic powder

2 tablespoons lime juice

1 1/2 tablespoon dill pickle relish

1 tablespoon dried onion flakes

1/2 teaspoon salt

Directions

Whisk together all the ingredients for the tartar sauce until well-combined. Chill for at least30 minutes until serving. Whisk eggs in a medium bowl. In another bowl, combine almond flour, cayenne pepper, basil, garlic, salt, and pepper. Dip fish sticks in egg, then flour mixture; coat well and place sticks in a plate. Heat 1/4 cup coconut oil in a large skillet over medium high heat. Add half of the fish sticks and cook for 2-3 minutes on each side until well-browned. Leave enough room around fish sticks so that they aren't overcrowded. Drain sticks on paper towels in a plate. Heat another 1/4 cup coconut oil and cook remaining half of the fish sticks. Serve with the prepared Garlic Lime Tartar Sauce.

Ingredients

1 pound lean chicken breast, skinless and boneless

2 tablespoons Stevia

1/4 cup Dijon mustard

1 tablespoon olive oil

1/4 cup rosemary leaves, roughly chopped

1 lemon, zested and juiced

1 tablespoon cayenne pepper

1/2 teaspoon ground black pepper

1/2 teaspoon sea salt

Directions

Place chicken breasts in a 7 x 11 inch baking dish.

Mix together all ingredients except the chicken, in a medium bowl. Pour prepared marinade over chicken;

turn sides to coat. Cover, place in fridge, and marinate for 15 minutes to 1 hour, or overnight for best flavor. Bake at 350°F for 18-20 minutes, or until internal temperature reaches 165°F. Pour extra sauce over top and serve.

Roasted Pork Tenderloin with Blueberry Sauce

Ingredients

1/2 teaspoon dried basil

1/2 teaspoon dried rosemary, crushed

1/4 teaspoon garlic powder

1/4 teaspoon dry mustard powder

1/8 teaspoon celery seed

1/8 teaspoon dried parsley

1/8 teaspoon cayenne pepper

1/2 teaspoon sea salt

1/2 teaspoon freshly ground black pepper

1-1/4 pound pork tenderloin

Blueberry sauce:

1 small onion, diced

1-1/2 cups frozen blueberries, thawed

1/4 cup apple cider vinegar

1 teaspoon raw honey

1/2 teaspoon dried thyme

1/2 teaspoon freshly ground black pepper

1/2 tablespoon olive oil

Directions

Preheat oven to 400 degrees F. Place pork in a roasting pan.

Combine first 9 ingredients in a small bowl and rub onto the pork. Roast for 25 minutes (or until internal temperature reaches 155° F).

In a small saucepan, sauté onion in olive oil over medium-high heat, about 5 minutes. Add the remaining sauce ingredients and cook for another 5 minutes, or until sauce is thickened. Pool sauce on serving plates and top with slices of roasted pork.

Carob Chip Cookies

Ingredients

3/4 cup raw honey

3/4 cup almond butter

2 1/4 cups almond flour

2 1/4 cups carob chocolate chips (chatfield's all natural carob chips)

1 teaspoon pure vanilla extract

1 teaspoon baking soda

1 teaspoon baking powder

1/2 teaspoon sea salt, or to taste

2 organic free-range eggs

1 teaspoon coconut oil (for greasing)

Directions

Preheat oven to 375 degrees F. Prepare a baking sheet and grease. In a medium bowl, mix gradually the almond butter, honey, eggs and vanilla. In a different bowl, sift the baking soda, gluten free flour mix, baking powder and salt. Mix in the butter mixture. Make sure to mix thoroughly. Finally, add the carob chips. Drop cookie mixture on the baking sheet 2 inches apart using a teaspoon. Place the baking sheet in the oven and bake for 8 minutes or until cookies turn to light brown. Let cool for 2 minutes and remove cookies from the baking sheet.

Gluten Free Almond Butter and Banana Sandwiches

Ingredients

1/4 cup coconut oil

1 cup almond nuts

10 drops liquid stevia (or raw honey)

Pinch of salt, or to taste

16 gluten free sliced breads

8 ripe bananas, sliced lengthwise

Directions

In a food processor, combine coconut oil, almond nuts, stevia, and salt thoroughly until it forms a butter paste. Let cool. Spread 2 tablespoons of almond butter on each pair of gluten free breads, add banana slices. Serve.

Citrus Berry Parfait

Ingredients

1 cup coconut butter, melted

1/2 cup organic low-fat lemon yogurt

1 cup fresh blackberries or blueberries

1 cup fresh raspberries or strawberries

2 tablespoons raw honey

1 cup walnuts or almonds, chopped

Directions

In a small bowl, mix together honey, lemon yogurt, and coconut butter and stir thoroughly.

In a separate bowl, combine the black berries and raspberries. Layer the berries and coconut butter mixture in parfait glasses and sprinkle walnuts on top.

Gluten-Free Chocolate Cupcakes

Ingredients

130 grams almond butter

130 grams Gluten-Free Self-Rising Flour

130 grams Gluten-Free vanilla powder

1 ½ tablespoon carob powder

½ tablespoon pure vanilla extract

3 tablespoons raw honey

2 organic free-range eggs

Icing:

100 grams almond butter

100grams stevia

Directions

Preheat oven to 190 degrees C. Line paper liners in a standard cupcake tin (12 cupcakes).

Whisk together the honey and butter in a medium bowl until fluffy and pale. Add the eggs, carob powder, and flour and blend well.

Place the mixture in the cupcake tin with the paper liners and bake for 20 minutes.

To prepare the icing, mix together the stevia and butter in a bowl until soft and light. In a piping bag, place the mixture of the stevia and butter. Spoon the icing on top of each cupcake.

Garbanzo Bean Chocolate Cake

Ingredients

1 1/2 cups gluten-free semisweet chocolate chips

5 tablespoons almond butter

1 (19 ounce) can garbanzo beans, rinsed and drained

4 eggs

3/4 cup unrefined brown sugar

1/2 teaspoon baking powder

1 tablespoon unsweetened cocoa powder

1 teaspoon pure vanilla extract

1 tablespoon coconut oil

Directions

Preheat the oven to 350 degrees F (175 degrees C). Grease a 9-inch round cake pan with coconut oil.

Place the chocolate chips and almond butter into a microwave-safe bowl. Cook in the microwave for about 2 minutes, or until melted and smooth.

Combine the beans and eggs in the bowl of a food processor, and process until smooth. Mix in the sugar and the baking powder, melted chocolate mixture, and vanilla; blend until smooth and well blended. Transfer the batter to the prepared cake pan.

Bake for 40 minutes, or until a toothpick inserted into the center of the cake comes out clean or with only a few crumbs sticking to it. Cool in the pan on a wire rack for 10-15 minutes. Invert onto a serving plate and dust with cocoa powder. Serve.

Poached Pears and Vanilla Ice Cream with Chocolate-Mango Sauce

Ingredients

1 cup organic mango nectar

1 cup dry white wine

1/2 cup unrefined brown sugar

4 slightly under-ripe pears, peeled, halved, cored

4 ounces semisweet chocolate, chopped

1 cup gluten-free low-fat vanilla ice cream

Directions

Mix together the pear nectar, white wine and sugar in large saucepan and bring to a boil over medium-high heat.

Add pears and turn heat to medium-low. Simmer covered for 8 minutes, or until pears are tender.

Using slotted spoon, transfer pear halves to individual plates, cut side up. Turn heat to medium-high. Boil poaching liquid for 8 minutes, or until syrupy and reduced by a quarter. Remove pan from heat. Whisk in chocolate until melted and sauce is smooth. Top each pear half with 2 tablespoons vanilla ice cream and drizzle with warm chocolate sauce.

Almond-stuffed Baked Apples with Almond Whipped Cream

Ingredients

6 apples

1/2 cup almond nuts, crushed

3 tablespoons raw honey

1/2 teaspoon nutmeg

1/4 teaspoon cinnamon

Zest of 2 small lemons

2 tablespoons almond butter

1 pinch sea salt

Almond Whipped Cream:

1 1/2 cups gluten-free low fat whipping cream

1 teaspoon pure almond extract

1/2 teaspoon ground nutmeg

1 teaspoon ground cinnamon

1 tablespoon raw honey

Directions

Preheat oven to 375 degrees.

Cut out the cores of the apple with a paring knife and trim about 1/2-inch slice from the bottom of each apple. Place cored apples in a baking dish and make them sit flat. Fill each apple with crushed almond nuts. Combine the honey, nutmeg, cinnamon, and lemon zest in a bowl and add to the stuffed apples. Stir together almond butter and salt. Top each apple with 1 teaspoon of almond butter mixture. Bake stuffed apples for 20–30 minutes. Transfer baked apples in serving plates. Combine all the whipped cream ingredients in a blender or food processor and process until smooth and creamy. Spoon 2 tablespoons of almond whipped cream on top of each stuffed apple.

Ingredients

1 1/2 cups fresh strawberries, sliced

1 cup fresh blueberries

1 cup fresh raspberries

1 lime, juiced

1 tablespoon raw honey

1 cup walnuts, chopped

Coconut Vanilla Ice Cream:

2 cups ice cold organic full-fat coconut milk

1/2 cup raw honey

2 teaspoons pure vanilla extract

Directions

Prepare the Coconut Vanilla Ice Cream: Combine coconut milk, honey, and vanilla in a blender. Cover and blend on High until smooth and frothy. Pour the liquid into a frozen ice cream bowl, cover, and start ice cream maker to churn it. Transfer to a freezer safe container; cover and serve.

Chill six parfait glasses.

Toss together the berries in a bowl and drizzle with honey and fresh lime juice.

Layer the berries, walnuts and coconut ice cream in parfait glasses.

Steamed Broccoli

Ingredients:

6 cups broccoli florets

Directions:

Pour 1½ cups water into the inner pot of the Instant Pot. Place a steam rack inside. Place the broccoli florets inside a steamer basket and place the basket on the steam rack. Steam within 1 minute. Remove the steamer basket and serve.

Boiled Cabbage

Ingredients:

1 large head green cabbage

3 cups vegetable broth

1 teaspoon salt

½ teaspoon black pepper

Directions:

Place the cabbage, broth, salt, and pepper in the inner pot. Cook within 5 minutes. Serve.

Vegetable "Cheese" Sauce

Ingredients:

1 small yellow onion, peeled and chopped

1 medium zucchini, peeled and sliced

6 cloves garlic, chopped

2¼ cups vegetable broth, divided

¼ teaspoon paprika

1 medium sweet potato, peeled and chopped

½ cup nutritional yeast

Directions:

Place the onion, zucchini, garlic, and ¼ cup broth into the inner pot. Press the Sauté button and let the vegetables sauté until soft, 5 minutes. Press the Cancel button. Add the remaining 2 cups broth, paprika, and sweet potato. Cook within 6 minutes. Allow to cool for a few minutes and then transfer the mixture to a large blender. Add the nutritional yeast to the blender with the other ingredients and blend on high until thoroughly combined and smooth. Serve warm as a topping for the vegetables of your choice.

Ingredients:

½ cup dry quinoa, 1 (10-ounce) bag frozen shelled edamame, 1 cup vegetable broth, ¼ cup reduced-sodium tamari, ¼ cup natural almond butter

3 tablespoons toasted sesame seed oil

½ teaspoon pure stevia powder

1 head purple cabbage, cored and chopped

Directions:

Place the quinoa, edamame, and broth in the inner pot of your Instant Pot. Cook within 2 minutes.

Whisk the tamari, almond butter, sesame seed oil, and stevia in a small bowl. Set aside. Fluff the quinoa using a fork, and then transfer the mixture to a large bowl. Allow the quinoa and edamame to cool, and then add the purple cabbage to the bowl and toss to combine. Put the dressing and toss again. Serve.

Ingredients:

1 large head cauliflower, cored and cut into large florets

Directions:

Put 2 cups water into the inner pot. Place a steam rack inside. Place the cauliflower inside a steamer basket and place the basket on the steam rack, steam within 2 minutes. Carefully remove the steamer basket and serve.

Ingredients:

1 tablespoon coconut oil

12 ounces Brussels sprouts, tough ends removed and cut in half

12 ounces carrots (about 4 medium), peeled, ends removed, and cut into 1' chunks

¼ cup fresh lime juice

¼ cup apple cider vinegar

½ cup coconut amino

¼ cup almond butter

Directions:

Sauté the Brussels sprouts and carrots and sauté until browned, about 5–7 minutes. While the vegetables are browning, make the sauce. Mix the lime juice, vinegar, coconut amino, and almond butter in a small bowl.

Pour the sauce over the vegetables—Cook within 6 minutes. Serve.

Lemony Cauliflower Rice

Ingredients:

1 tablespoon avocado oil

1 small yellow onion, peeled and diced

1 teaspoon minced garlic

4 cups riced cauliflower

Juice from 1 little lemon

½ teaspoon salt

¼ teaspoon black pepper

Directions:

Put the oil to the pot, and heat 1 minute. Add the onion and sauté 5 minutes. Add the garlic and sauté 1 more minute. Add the cauliflower rice, lemon juice, salt, and pepper and stir to combine—Cook within 1 minute. Transfer to a bowl for serving.

Ingredients:

1-pound asparagus, woody ends removed

Juice from ½ large lemon

¼ teaspoon kosher salt

Directions:

Add ½ cup water to the inner pot and add the steam rack. Add the asparagus to the steamer basket and place the basket on top of the rack, then steam within 1 minute. Transfer, and top with lemon juice and salt.

Lemon Garlic Red Chard

Ingredients:

1 tablespoon avocado oil

1 small yellow onion, peeled and diced

1 bunch red chard, leaves and stems chopped and kept separate (about 12 ounces)

3 cloves garlic, minced

¾ teaspoon salt

Juice from ½ medium lemon

1 teaspoon lemon zest

Directions:

Put the oil to the inner pot and allow it to heat 1 minute. Add the onion and chard stems and sauté 5 minutes. Put the garlic and sauté another 30 seconds. Put the chard leaves, salt, and lemon juice and stir to combine. Turn off. Cook again within 60 seconds. Scoop the chard mixture into a serving bowl and top with lemon zest.

Lemon Ginger Broccoli and Carrots

Ingredients:

1 tablespoon avocado oil

1' fresh ginger, peeled and thinly sliced

1 clove garlic, minced

2 broccoli crowns, florets

2 large carrots, sliced

½ teaspoon kosher salt

Juice from ½ large lemon

¼ cup of water

Directions:

Put the oil to the inner pot. Heat-up within 2 minutes. Add the ginger and garlic and sauté 1 minute. Add the broccoli, carrots, and salt and stir to combine. Turn off. Add the lemon juice and water and use a wooden spoon to scrape up any brown bits—Cook within 2 minutes. Serve immediately.

Curried Mustard Greens

Ingredients:

1 tablespoon avocado oil, 1 medium white onion, peeled and chopped, 1 tablespoon peeled and chopped ginger, 3 cloves garlic, minced, 2 tablespoons curry powder, ½ teaspoon salt,¼ teaspoon black

pepper, 2 cups vegetable broth, ½ cup coconut cream, 1 large bunch mustard greens, chopped

Directions:

Add the oil to the inner pot. Press the Sauté button and heat the oil 2 minutes. Sauté the onion within 5 minutes. Add the ginger, garlic, curry, salt, and pepper and sauté 1 more minute. Stir in the vegetable broth and coconut cream until combined and then allow it to come to a boil, about 2–3 minutes more. Turn off. Stir in the mustard greens until everything is well combined. Cook within 60 seconds. Transfer to a bowl and serve.

"Cheesy" Brussels Sprouts and Carrots

Ingredients:

1-pound Brussels sprouts, tough ends removed and cut in half

1-pound baby carrots

1 cup chicken stock

2 tablespoons lemon juice

½ cup nutritional yeast

¼ teaspoon salt

Directions:

Add the Brussels sprouts, carrots, stock, lemon juice, nutritional yeast, and salt to the inner pot. Stir well to combine. Cook within 10 minutes.
Transfer the vegetables and sauce to a bowl and serve.

Garlic Green Beans

Ingredients:

12 ounces green beans, ends trimmed

4 cloves garlic, minced

1 tablespoon avocado oil

½ teaspoon salt

1 cup of water

Directions:

Place the green beans in a medium bowl and toss with the garlic, oil, and salt. Transfer this mixture to the steamer basket. Put one cup of water into the pot and put the steam rack inside. Place the steamer basket with the green beans on top of the steam rack—Cook within 5 minutes. Transfer to a bowl for serving.

Simple Beet Salad

Ingredients:

6 medium beets, peeled and cut into small cubes

1 cup of water

¼ cup extra-virgin olive oil

¼ cup apple cider vinegar

1 teaspoon Dijon mustard

¼ teaspoon pure stevia powder

½ teaspoon salt

¼ teaspoon black pepper

1 large shallot, peeled and diced

1 large stalk celery, ends removed and thinly sliced

Directions:

Place the beets into the steamer basket. Put 1 cup water into the inner pot and place the steam rack inside. Place the steamer basket with the beets on top of the steam rack. Meanwhile, in a small container or jar with a tight lid, add the oil, vinegar, mustard, stevia, salt, and pepper and shake well to combine. Set aside. Cook within 5 minutes. Remove, and let the beets cool completely. Place the shallot and celery in a large bowl and then add the cooked, cooled beets. Serve with the dressing and toss to coat.

Cabbage and Avocado Salsa

Ingredients:

¼ cup veggie stock

2 tablespoons olive oil

2 spring onions, chopped

1 red cabbage head, shredded

1 avocado, peeled, pitted, and cubed

Directions:

Add tomatoes and all other ingredients to a suitable cooking pot. Cover the pot's lid and cook for 12 minutes on medium heat. Serve fresh and enjoy.

Spinach Cabbage Slaw

Ingredients:

2 cups red cabbage, shredded

1 tablespoon mayonnaise

1 spring onion, chopped

1-lb. baby spinach

½ cup chicken stock

Directions:

Start by adding onion to a suitable pan, to sauté for 2 minutes.

Add spinach, stock and mayonnaise then mix well.

Serve fresh and enjoy.

Chicken Pesto Salad

Ingredients:

1-lb. chicken breast, skinless, boneless, and cubed

2 tablespoons basil pesto

2 tablespoons olive oil

2 tablespoons garlic, chopped

1 cup tomatoes, crushed

Directions:

Start by adding oil, chicken, and garlic to a cooking pan.

Then sauté for 5 minutes. Stir in pesto and tomatoes.

Cover the pot's lid and cook for 15 minutes on medium

heat. Serve fresh and enjoy.

Ingredients:

1 and ½ lbs. mixed bell peppers, cut into strips

1 tablespoon avocado oil

½ cup tomato passata

1 avocado, peeled, pitted, and cubed

Salt and black pepper, to taste

Directions:

Add bell peppers and all other ingredients to a suitable cooking pot. Cover the pot's lid and cook for 12 minutes on medium heat. Serve fresh and enjoy.

Ingredients:

1-lb. salmon fillets, boneless, skinless, and cubed

Salt and black pepper, to taste

¼ lb. Swiss chard, torn

1 spring onion, chopped

¼ cup chicken stock

Directions:

Add chard with all other ingredients to a cooking pot. Cover the pot's lid and cook for 15 minutes on medium heat. Use an immersion blender to blend the spread until smooth. Serve fresh and enjoy.

Olives Coconut Dip

Ingredients:

4 cups baby spinach

½ cup coconut cream

Salt and black pepper, to taste

4 garlic cloves, roasted and minced

1 cup kalamata olives, pitted and halved

Directions:

Add olives and all other ingredients to a cooking pot. Cover the pot's lid and cook for 10 minutes on medium heat.

Use an immersion blender to blend the olives mixture until smooth. Serve fresh and enjoy.

Ingredients:

3 shallots, minced

1 and ½ lbs. mixed peppers, roughly chopped

¼ cup chicken stock

1 tablespoon olive oil

2 tablespoons basil, chopped

Directions:

Start by sautéing shallots with oil in a pan, then sauté for 2 minutes. Stir in remaining ingredients and mix well Cover the pot's lid and cook for 13 minutes on medium heat. Use an immersion blender to blend the pepper mixture until smooth Serve fresh and enjoy.

Ingredients:

1 bunch watercress, trimmed

¼ cup chicken stock

1 cup tomato, cubed

1 avocado, peeled, pitted, and cubed

2 zucchinis, cubed

Directions:

Start by adding watercress and all other ingredients to a cooking pot. Cover the pot's lid and cook for 10 minutes on medium heat. Serve fresh and enjoy.

Ingredients:

1 tablespoon lime juice

2 tablespoons avocado oil

1-lb. beef stew meat, cubed

2 garlic cloves, minced

1 cup beef stock

Directions:

Start by adding oil and meat to a cooking pan, then sauté for 5 minutes. Stir in remaining ingredients and mix well Cover the pot's lid and cook for 30 minutes on medium heat. Serve fresh and enjoy

Olives Parsley Spread

Ingredients:

2 cups black olives, pitted and halved

2 garlic cloves, minced

1 tablespoon lemon juice

1 tablespoon olive oil

¼ cup chicken stock

Salt and black pepper, to taste

Directions:

Add black olive, chicken stock, and all other ingredients to a suitable cooking pot. Cover the pot's lid and cook for 10 minutes on medium heat. Blend this mixture using a handheld blender. Serve fresh and enjoy.

Basic Mushroom Salsa

Ingredients:

1-lb. white mushrooms halved

¼ cup chicken stock

1 tablespoon basil, chopped

2 tomatoes, cubed

1 avocado, peeled, pitted, and cubed

Salt and black pepper, to taste

Directions:

Add mushrooms and all other ingredients to a suitable cooking pot. Cover the pot's lid and cook for 10 minutes on medium heat. Serve fresh and enjoy.

Ingredients:

1-lb. okra, trimmed

½ lb. shrimp, peeled and deveined

2 tablespoons olive oil

1 cup tomato passata, chopped

1 tablespoon cilantro, chopped

Salt and black pepper, to taste

Directions:

Add shrimp, okra, and all other ingredients to a suitable cooking pot. Cover the pot's lid and cook for 12 minutes on medium heat. Serve fresh and enjoy.

Thyme Celery Spread

Ingredients:

2 lbs. eggplant, roughly chopped

2 celery stalks, chopped

2 tablespoons olive oil

4 garlic cloves, minced

½ cup veggie stock

Salt and black pepper, to taste

Directions:

Stat by adding oil, celery stalks, and garlic to a pan, then sauté for 2 minutes. Stir in remaining ingredients and mix well Cover the pot's lid and cook for 10 minutes on medium heat. Blend the spread using an immersion blender until smooth Serve fresh and enjoy.

Nutmeg Spiced Endives

Ingredients:

4 endives, trimmed and halved

Salt and black pepper to the taste

2 tablespoons olive oil

1 teaspoon nutmeg, ground

1 tablespoon chives, chopped

Directions:

Toss endives with all other ingredients in a baking sheet. Bake the endives for 5 minutes in a preheated oven at 350 degrees F. Serve fresh and enjoy.

Ingredients:

1 cucumber, peeled and shredded

1 garlic clove, minced

2 Tablespoons chopped fresh dill

1 teaspoon salt

1 cup plain coconut yogurt

2 Tablespoons freshly squeezed lemon juice

2 Tablespoons extra-virgin olive oil

1 scallion, chopped

Directions:

Set down the shredded cucumber in a big sieve to drain.

Take a small bowl and stir together the garlic, salt, yogurt, scallion, dill, and lemon juice. Fold in the dried cucumber and take to a serving bowl. Before serving, sprinkle with olive oil.

Ingredients:

1 can white beans

1 Tablespoon tahini, or almond butter

¼ cup chopped pitted green olives

1 garlic clove, 1 Tablespoon chopped fresh parsley

¼ Teaspoon salt, 2 Tablespoons freshly squeezed lemon juice, 3 Tablespoons extra-virgin olive oil

Directions:

Take a food processor and mix the white beans, garlic, and tahini. With the machine in low-power mode, carefully add the olive oil in a thin, stable stream.

Add the parsley, olives, and salt. Pulse to combine. Pour in the lemon juice. Take to a serving bowl and serve along with raw vegetables

Mashed Avocado with Jicama Slices

Ingredients:

2 ripe avocados, pitted

1 scallion, sliced

2 Tablespoons chopped fresh cilantro

½ Teaspoon ground turmeric

Juice of ½ lemon

1 teaspoon salt

¼ Teaspoon freshly ground black pepper

1 jicama, peeled and cut into ¼-inch-thick slices

Directions:

Take a small bowl and mix the scooped-out avocado, turmeric, the scallion, cilantro, lemon juice, salt, and pepper.

Mash the ingredients together until mixed and still somewhat chunky. Serve along with jicama slices.

Creamy Broccoli Dip

Ingredients:

1 cup broccoli florets

1 garlic clove

½ avocado

1 Tablespoon freshly squeezed lemon juice

1 teaspoon salt

¾ cup unsweetened almond yogurt or coconut yogurt

½ Teaspoon dried dill

Pinch red pepper flakes

1 scallion, coarsely chopped

Directions:

Fill two inches of water in a pot, place it over medium flame, and set a steamer basket. Put the broccoli on the steamer basket, cover, and let it steam for five minutes, or until the broccoli attains a bright green hue. Take off the pan of the flame and drain the broccoli. Take a food processor and add the garlic, avocado, dill, scallion, yogurt, lemon juice, salt, and red pepper flakes. Pulse a few times until the mixture seems to be chopped. Add the broccoli and process until appropriately blended but not entirely puréed. Serve along with Sweet Potato Chips or chopped fresh vegetables such as carrots and celery.

Smoked Trout and Mango Wraps

Ingredients:

4 ounces smoked trout, divided

1 cup chopped mango, divided

4 large green-leaf lettuce leaves, thick stems removed

1 scallion, sliced, divided

2 Tablespoons freshly squeezed lemon juice, divided

Directions:

Find a flat surface and place lettuce leaves on it. Put pieces of trout and mango over each leaf equally. Dust with the scallions and sprinkle with the lemon juice. Wrap the lettuce leaves in burrito style and set them seam-side down on a serving platter

Kale Chips

Ingredients:

1 bunch kale, thoroughly washed and dried, ribs detached, and cut into two-inch strips

2 Tablespoons extra-virgin olive oil

1 teaspoon of sea salt

Directions:

Power on the oven and heat it to 275°F. In a large bowl, bare hands mix the kale and olive oil until the kale gets consistently coated with the oil.

Take the kale to a baking sheet, spreading it in a layer dust with the sea salt. Bake within 20 minutes. Turn the side of the chips halfway through the banking process, so both sides attain the crispiness. Cool the chips a bit before you serve.

Ingredients:

8 thin slices smoked turkey

1 cup packed arugula, divided

Pinch salt

2 zucchinis, quartered lengthwise

Directions:

Place a single slice of smoked turkey on an active working surface. Top with one zucchini stick, one-fourth cup of arugula, and dust of salt. Wrap the turkey all over the vegetables and lay it on a serving dish seam-side down. Repeat for the remaining ingredients. Cover and chill until ready to serve.

Ingredients:

1 can drained chickpeas (15 ounces)

½ Teaspoon ground cumin

½ Teaspoon ground turmeric

½ Teaspoon chipotle powder

1 teaspoon salt

¼ Teaspoon garlic powder

½ Teaspoon onion powder

2 Tablespoons extra-virgin olive oil

Directions:

Power on the oven and heat it to 375°F. Make the drained chickpeas dry using a paper towel. Mix the salt, chipotle powder, onion powder, cumin, turmeric, and garlic powder in a small bowl. Take a medium bowl and combine the dry chickpeas and olive oil. Softly stir the chickpeas to place over a coat of oil. Dust the salt mixture over the chickpeas. Stir the combo till coated evenly. Take a large baking sheet, raise its sides (to prevent the chickpeas from falling off the sheet), and spread the chickpeas all over layer-wise. Lay down the sheet in the preheated oven and bake for thirty to forty minutes, stirring in between, or until the chickpeas are dry and crunchy. Cool entirely before eating.

Sweet Potato Chips

Ingredients:

3 Tablespoons extra-virgin olive oil

1 teaspoon of sea salt

2 larges thinly sliced sweet potatoes

Directions:

Power on the oven and heat it to 250°F. Place the rack in the center of the oven.

Take a large bowl and drop in the sweet potatoes' slices along with olive oil. Arrange the slices individually on 2 baking sheets dust with the sea salt. Lay the sheets inside the preheated oven and bake for about two hours; make sure to rotate the pans and flip the chips after 45 – 60 minutes. As soon as the chips turn light brown and attain the crispiness, take them off the oven. Some may be a bit mushy, but they will again turn crisp as they begin to cool. Let the chips cool for about ten minutes before serving. Serve straight away. The chips will again turn mushy after a few hours.

Mini Snack Muffins

Ingredients:

¼ cup extra-virgin olive oil

1 cup brown rice flour

1 cup canned pumpkin

¼ Tablespoon olive oil for greasing

1 Tablespoon baking powder

½ Teaspoon salt

1 teaspoon ground cinnamon

4 eggs

1 cup almond flour

1 cup shredded carrot

Directions:

Power on the oven and heat it to 375°F.

With a small brush, line a mini muffin tin with either cupcake liners or little olive oil.

Take a medium bowl and combine the almond flour, baking powder, brown rice flour, salt, and cinnamon.

Add the carrot, eggs, pumpkin, and olive oil. Stir until everything blends properly.

Scoop the batter in each muffin cup, filling each three-quarter only.

Lay the tin inside the preheated oven and bake for fifteen minutes, or until the muffins turn slightly brown.

Take off of the oven and let it cool for ten minutes before removing the muffins from the tin.

Ingredients:

2 cup frozen unsweetened strawberries, thawed

1 (15-ounce) can coconut milk

1 Tablespoon chia seeds

1 Tablespoon freshly squeezed lemon juice

1 teaspoon vanilla extract

Directions:

Arrange six ice pop molds or prepare per the manufacturer's guidelines.

Take a medium bowl and stir together the chia seeds, strawberries, lemon juice, coconut milk, and vanilla.

Allow the mixture to lay still for five minutes, so the chia seeds thicken slightly.

Consistently divide the mixture amongst the molds. Place one ice pop stick in every mold. Freeze the pops for approximately five hours, or overnight. Serve.

Ingredients:

2 Tablespoons extra-virgin olive oil

4 cups broccoli florets

2 Tablespoons toasted sesame seeds

1 Tablespoon grated fresh ginger

¼Teaspoon sea salt

1 teaspoon sesame oil

2 garlic cloves, minced

Directions:

Heat-up the olive oil and sesame oil in a non-stick pan over medium flame until they start to shimmer. Now add the broccoli, ginger, and salt. Cook within 7 minutes, frequently stirring, until the broccoli begins attaining a brown hue. Add the garlic. Cook for thirty seconds, stirring continually. Take off of the heat and stir the sesame seeds.

Dill and Salmon Pâté

Ingredients:

six ounces cooked salmon, bones and skin removed

1 Tablespoon chopped fresh dill, ½ Teaspoon sea salt

¼ cup heavy (whipping) cream

Directions:

Take a blender or a food processor (or instead a large bowl using a mixer), mix the lemon zest, salmon, heavy cream, dill, and salt. Blend till you attain the proper consistency for the smoothie.

Chickpea - Garlic Hummus

Ingredients:

3 garlic cloves, minced

2 Tablespoons tahini

1 can chickpeas, drained

2 Tablespoons extra-virgin olive oil

juice of 1 lemon

½ Teaspoon sea salt

paprika, for garnishing

Directions:

Mix the garlic, tahini, olive oil, chickpeas, lemon juice, and salt in a blender. Blend till you attain the proper consistency for the snack. Garnish as desired.

Sautéed Apples, Ginger, and Cinnamon

Ingredients:

2 Tablespoons coconut oil

3 apples, peeled and sliced

1 teaspoon ground cinnamon

1 packet stevia

1 Tablespoon grated fresh ginger

pinch sea salt

Directions:

Heat-up the coconut oil in a non-stick pan over medium flame. Add the apples, cinnamon, ginger, stevia, and salt. Cook for seven to ten minutes, stirring in between until the apples turn mushy.

Conclusion

Leaky gut is not a recognized diagnosis at this time, but it describes the phenomenon of increased intestinal permeability that is sometimes associated with certain gastrointestinal symptoms and illnesses. Proponents of leaky gut syndrome suggest that an association exists with autoimmune conditions, neuropsychiatric conditions, and some nonspecific symptoms such as abdominal bloating, fatigue, headaches, and joint pain.

There is no standard diagnostic test for leaky gut. In general, gut health can be supported by eating a balanced diet, limiting alcohol intake, and managing stress, among other lifestyle factors.